RENAL DIET FOR BEGINNERS

Easy, Delicious Recipes to Manage Your Kidney Health

Dr Lily Morgan

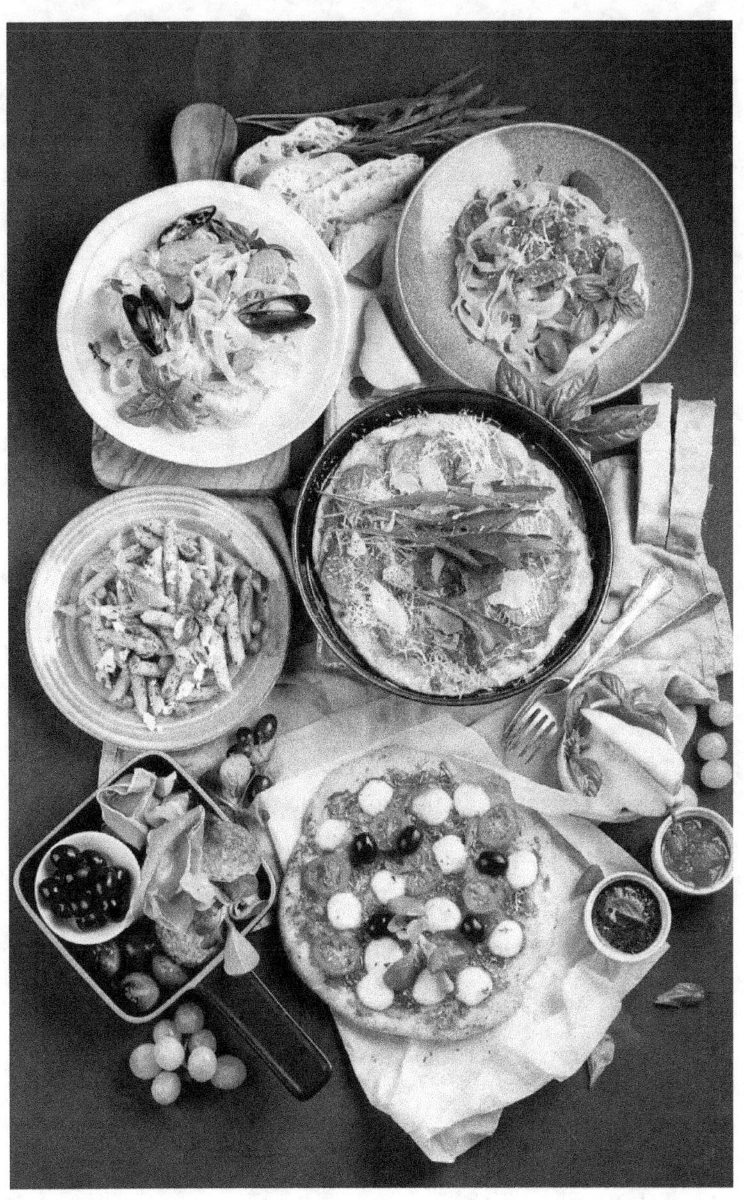

TABLE OF CONTENTS

INTRODUCTION **9**

Why Is a Renal Diet Important? 9

Tips for Success on the Renal Diet: 10

Chapter 1: 30 Day Meal Plan **12**

Week 1: 12

Week 2: 14

Week 3: 16

Week 4: 19

Chapter 2: Breakfast Recipes **23**

Low-Sodium Oatmeal with Berries 23

Scrambled Egg Whites with Spinach 24

Yogurt Parfait with Nuts and Honey 24

Vegetable Frittata 25

Rice Pudding with Cinnamon 26

Banana Walnut Pancakes 26

Smoothie with Kale and Blueberries 27

Breakfast Burrito with Beans 27

Quinoa Porridge with Almonds 28

Greek Yogurt and Fruit Bowl 29

Cereal with Fresh Fruit 29

Spinach and Mushroom Omelette 30

Whole Grain Waffles 30

Avocado Toast with Tomatoes 31

Cottage Cheese and Pineapple 31

Breakfast Tacos with Salsa 32

Sweet Potato Hash 32

Bran Muffins 33

Chapter 3: Lunch Recipes.................................... 34

Grilled Chicken Salad 34

Tuna and White Bean Salad....................................... 35

Quinoa and Vegetable Bowl 36

Turkey and Avocado Wrap... 36

Lentil Soup... 37

Spinach and Chickpea Salad...................................... 38

Brown Rice and Veggie Stir-fry 39

Salmon Salad with Dill Dressing............................... 40

Minestrone Soup 41

Shrimp and Broccoli Stir-fry 42

Black Bean and Corn Salad 42

Chicken and Rice Bowl 43

Egg Salad Sandwich 44

Vegetable and Barley Soup.. 45

Caprese Salad... 46

Pita Bread with Hummus.. 46

Baked Sweet Potato with Beans 47

Veggie Wrap with Greek Yogurt Sauce 48

Chapter 4: Dinner Recipes 49

Baked Salmon with Asparagus 49

Lemon Herb Grilled Chicken... 50

Stuffed Bell Peppers 51

Eggplant Parmesan.. 51

Beef and Vegetable Stir-fry 52

Spaghetti Squash with Tomato Sauce............................ 53

Teriyaki Tofu and Broccoli... 54

Pork Tenderloin with Apples 55

Baked Cod with Lemon and Herbs 56

Quinoa-Stuffed Portobello Mushrooms........................ 56

Veggie and Chickpea Curry.. 57

Turkey Meatloaf.. 58

Ratatouille 58

Cilantro Lime Shrimp 59

Roasted Vegetable Platter 60

Baked Ziti with Ricotta... 60

BBQ Tofu Skewers 61

Beef and Bean Chili.. 61

Chapter 5: Snacks and Appetizers 63

Guacamole with Veggie Sticks...................................... 63

Mixed Nuts.. 64

Hummus and Whole Wheat Pita.................................... 65

Greek Yogurt Dip with Cucumbers 65

Sliced Apple with Almond Butter................................ 66

Popcorn Seasoned with Herbs 66

Cottage Cheese with Peaches.................................... 67

Deviled Eggs 68

Edamame with Sea Salt 68

Cherry Tomato Bruschetta.. 69

Trail Mix with Dried Fruit 70

Baked Sweet Potato Fries 70

Salsa and Baked Tortilla Chips................................. 71

Mini Caprese Skewers 72

Spinach and Artichoke Dip....................................... 72

Roasted Red Pepper Hummus 73

Stuffed Mushrooms.. 74

Avocado Slices with Lime 75

Chapter 6: Desserts 76

Baked Apples with Cinnamon 76

Berry Parfait with Greek Yogurt................................ 77

Chocolate Avocado Mousse 77

Rice Pudding with Raisins....................................... 78

Banana Ice Cream 79

Lemon Sorbet... 79

Peach and Berry Crisp 80

Oatmeal Cookies with Raisins.................................... 81

Angel Food Cake with Berries 81

Pumpkin Pie with Oat Crust 82

Frozen Yogurt with Mango 83

Chia Seed Pudding 83

Poached Pears in Red Wine 84

Almond and Cherry Biscotti 85

Carrot Cake Bites 86

Pineapple Sorbet 87

Fig and Walnut Bars 87

Chocolate-Dipped Strawberries 88

CONCLUSION **90**

INTRODUCTION

T he Renal Diet, often referred to as a kidney-friendly diet, is a specialized nutritional plan designed to support individuals with kidney disease. It revolves around careful management of certain nutrients to reduce the workload on the kidneys while maintaining overall health.

Why Is a Renal Diet Important?

The significance of the Renal Diet lies in its ability to alleviate stress on the kidneys. For those with kidney issues, the organs may struggle to filter waste products and excess fluids effectively. The Renal Diet aims to minimize the accumulation of waste in the body, thus easing the burden on the kidneys. This diet can also help control blood pressure, manage electrolyte imbalances, and maintain overall well-being.

Tips for Success on the Renal Diet:

1. **Monitor Sodium Intake**: Sodium can cause fluid retention and elevate blood pressure. Limit high-sodium foods like processed meats, canned soups, and salty snacks.

2. **Watch Protein Consumption**: While protein is essential, excessive protein intake can strain the kidneys. Opt for high-quality, low-quantity protein sources such as lean meats, poultry, fish, and plant-based options.

3. **Control Phosphorus:** Phosphorus levels should be managed since high levels can weaken bones. Avoid foods rich in phosphorus, like dairy products and certain processed foods.

4. **Stay Hydrated:** Maintain proper hydration, but be cautious not to overhydrate. Your dietitian can help determine the right fluid balance for you.

5. **Manage Potassium:** Potassium levels should be regulated as imbalances can lead to heart problems. Choose low-potassium fruits and vegetables and follow your dietitian's recommendations.

6. **Limit Phosphorus Binders:** If prescribed, take phosphorus binders as directed by your healthcare provider to control phosphorus absorption.

7. **Regular Monitoring:** Regularly monitor your kidney function through blood tests. Adjust your diet as needed based on these results.

8. **Balanced Diet:** Focus on a well-balanced diet that includes a variety of foods to ensure you get essential nutrients without overloading the kidneys.

9. **Medication Adherence**: If your doctor has prescribed medications, take them as directed to manage underlying kidney conditions effectively.

Remember, the Renal Diet is highly individualized, and adherence is key to managing kidney health. Always consult with your healthcare team for personalized guidance on your renal diet journey.

Chapter 1: 30 Day Meal Plan

Week 1:

Day 1:

- Breakfast: Low-Sodium Oatmeal with Berries
- Lunch: Grilled Chicken Salad
- Dinner: Baked Salmon with Asparagus
- Snacks: Guacamole with Veggie Sticks
- Dessert: Baked Apples with Cinnamon

Day 2:

- Breakfast: Scrambled Egg Whites with Spinach
- Lunch: Tuna and White Bean Salad
- Dinner: Lemon Herb Grilled Chicken
- Snacks: Mixed Nuts
- Dessert: Berry Parfait with Greek Yogurt

Day 3:

- Breakfast: Yogurt Parfait with Nuts and Honey
- Lunch: Quinoa and Vegetable Bowl
- Dinner: Stuffed Bell Peppers

- Snacks: Hummus and Whole Wheat Pita
- Dessert: Chocolate Avocado Mousse

Day 4:

- Breakfast: Vegetable Frittata
- Lunch: Turkey and Avocado Wrap
- Dinner: Eggplant Parmesan
- Snacks: Greek Yogurt Dip with Cucumbers
- Dessert: Rice Pudding with Raisins

Day 5:

- Breakfast: Rice Pudding with Cinnamon
- Lunch: Lentil Soup
- Dinner: Beef and Vegetable Stir-fry
- Snacks: Sliced Apple with Almond Butter
- Dessert: Banana Ice Cream

Day 6:

- Breakfast: Banana Walnut Pancakes
- Lunch: Spinach and Chickpea Salad
- Dinner: Spaghetti Squash with Tomato Sauce
- Snacks: Popcorn Seasoned with Herbs

- Dessert: Lemon Sorbet

Day 7:

- Breakfast: Smoothie with Kale and Blueberries
- Lunch: Brown Rice and Veggie Stir-fry
- Dinner: Teriyaki Tofu and Broccoli
- Snacks: Cottage Cheese with Peaches
- Dessert: Peach and Berry Crisp

Week 2:

Day 8:

- Breakfast: Breakfast Burrito with Beans
- Lunch: Salmon Salad with Dill Dressing
- Dinner: Pork Tenderloin with Apples
- Snacks: Deviled Eggs
- Dessert: Oatmeal Cookies with Raisins

Day 9:

- Breakfast: Quinoa Porridge with Almonds
- Lunch: Minestrone Soup
- Dinner: Baked Cod with Lemon and Herbs
- Snacks: Edamame with Sea Salt

- Dessert: Angel Food Cake with Berries

Day 10:

- Breakfast: Greek Yogurt and Fruit Bowl
- Lunch: Shrimp and Broccoli Stir-fry
- Dinner: Quinoa-Stuffed Portobello Mushrooms
- Snacks: Cherry Tomato Bruschetta
- Dessert: Pumpkin Pie with Oat Crust

Day 11:

- Breakfast: Cereal with Fresh Fruit
- Lunch: Black Bean and Corn Salad
- Dinner: Veggie and Chickpea Curry
- Snacks: Trail Mix with Dried Fruit
- Dessert: Frozen Yogurt with Mango

Day 12:

- Breakfast: Spinach and Mushroom Omelette
- Lunch: Chicken and Rice Bowl
- Dinner: Turkey Meatloaf
- Snacks: Baked Sweet Potato Fries
- Dessert: Chia Seed Pudding

Day 13:

- Breakfast: Whole Grain Waffles
- Lunch: Egg Salad Sandwich
- Dinner: Ratatouille
- Snacks: Salsa and Baked Tortilla Chips
- Dessert: Poached Pears in Red Wine

Day 14:

- Breakfast: Avocado Toast with Tomatoes
- Lunch: Vegetable and Barley Soup
- Dinner: Cilantro Lime Shrimp
- Snacks: Mini Caprese Skewers
- Dessert: Almond and Cherry Biscotti

Week 3:

Day 15:

- Breakfast: Sweet Potato Hash
- Lunch: Caprese Salad
- Dinner: Roasted Vegetable Platter
- Snacks: Spinach and Artichoke Dip
- Dessert: Carrot Cake Bites

Day 16:

- Breakfast: Bran Muffins
- Lunch: Pita Bread with Hummus
- Dinner: Baked Ziti with Ricotta
- Snacks: Roasted Red Pepper Hummus
- Dessert: Pineapple Sorbet

Day 17:

- Breakfast: Cottage Cheese and Pineapple
- Lunch: Baked Sweet Potato with Beans
- Dinner: BBQ Tofu Skewers
- Snacks: Stuffed Mushrooms
- Dessert: Fig and Walnut Bars

Day 18:

- Breakfast: Breakfast Tacos with Salsa
- Lunch: Veggie Wrap with Greek Yogurt Sauce
- Dinner: Beef and Bean Chili
- Snacks: Avocado Slices with Lime
- Dessert: Chocolate-Dipped Strawberries

Day 19:

- Breakfast: Low-Sodium Oatmeal with Berries
- Lunch: Grilled Chicken Salad
- Dinner: Baked Salmon with Asparagus
- Snacks: Guacamole with Veggie Sticks
- Dessert: Baked Apples with Cinnamon

Day 20:

- Breakfast: Scrambled Egg Whites with Spinach
- Lunch: Tuna and White Bean Salad
- Dinner: Lemon Herb Grilled Chicken
- Snacks: Mixed Nuts
- Dessert: Berry Parfait with Greek Yogurt

Day 21:

- Breakfast: Yogurt Parfait with Nuts and Honey
- Lunch: Quinoa and Vegetable Bowl
- Dinner: Stuffed Bell Peppers
- Snacks: Hummus and Whole Wheat Pita
- Dessert: Chocolate Avocado Mousse

Week 4:

Day 22:

- Breakfast: Vegetable Frittata
- Lunch: Turkey and Avocado Wrap
- Dinner: Eggplant Parmesan
- Snacks: Greek Yogurt Dip with Cucumbers
- Dessert: Rice Pudding with Raisins

Day 23:

- Breakfast: Rice Pudding with Cinnamon
- Lunch: Lentil Soup
- Dinner: Beef and Vegetable Stir-fry
- Snacks: Sliced Apple with Almond Butter
- Dessert: Banana Ice Cream

Day 24:

- Breakfast: Banana Walnut Pancakes
- Lunch: Spinach and Chickpea Salad
- Dinner: Spaghetti Squash with Tomato Sauce
- Snacks: Popcorn Seasoned with Herbs
- Dessert: Lemon Sorbet

Day 25:

- Breakfast: Smoothie with Kale and Blueberries
- Lunch: Brown Rice and Veggie Stir-fry
- Dinner: Teriyaki Tofu and Broccoli
- Snacks: Cottage Cheese with Peaches
- Dessert: Peach and Berry Crisp

Day 26:

- Breakfast: Breakfast Burrito with Beans
- Lunch: Salmon Salad with Dill Dressing
- Dinner: Pork Tenderloin with Apples
- Snacks: Deviled Eggs
- Dessert: Oatmeal Cookies with Raisins

Day 27:

- Breakfast: Quinoa Porridge with Almonds
- Lunch: Minestrone Soup
- Dinner: Baked Cod with Lemon and Herbs
- Snacks: Edamame with Sea Salt
- Dessert: Angel Food Cake with Berries

Day 28:

- Breakfast: Greek Yogurt and Fruit Bowl
- Lunch: Shrimp and Broccoli Stir-fry
- Dinner: Quinoa-Stuffed Portobello Mushrooms
- Snacks: Cherry Tomato Bruschetta
- Dessert: Pumpkin Pie with Oat Crust

Day 29:

- Breakfast: Cereal with Fresh Fruit
- Lunch: Black Bean and Corn Salad
- Dinner: Veggie and Chickpea Curry
- Snacks: Trail Mix with Dried Fruit
- Dessert: Frozen Yogurt with Mango

Day 30:

- Breakfast: Spinach and Mushroom Omelette
- Lunch: Chicken and Rice Bowl
- Dinner: Turkey Meatloaf
- Snacks: Baked Sweet Potato Fries
- Dessert: Chia Seed Pudding

This completes the 30-day meal plan, providing a wide variety of renal-friendly recipes for each day of the month.

Chapter 2: Breakfast Recipes

In this chapter, we'll explore a delicious array of breakfast options designed with your renal health in mind. Each recipe is crafted to be both nutritious and flavorful, ensuring a great start to your day. Let's dive into these wholesome breakfast ideas:

Low-Sodium Oatmeal with Berries

Ingredients:

- 1/2 cup rolled oats
- 1 cup unsweetened almond milk
- 1/2 cup mixed berries
- 1 tablespoon honey (optional)

Instructions:

1. Combine oats and almond milk in a saucepan.
2. Cook over low heat, stirring, until oatmeal thickens.
3. Serve hot, topped with mixed berries and a drizzle of honey if desired.

Scrambled Egg Whites with Spinach

Ingredients:

- 3 egg whites
- 1/2 cup fresh spinach leaves
- Salt and pepper to taste

Instructions:

1. Whisk egg whites in a bowl and season with salt and pepper.
2. In a non-stick pan, sauté spinach until wilted.
3. Pour in egg whites and scramble until cooked through.

Yogurt Parfait with Nuts and Honey

Ingredients:

- 1/2 cup low-fat yogurt
- 1/4 cup chopped nuts (almonds, walnuts)
- 1 tablespoon honey
- 1/4 cup fresh fruit (e.g., berries)

Instructions:

1. Layer yogurt, nuts, and honey in a glass.
2. Top with fresh fruit.
3. Enjoy the creamy and crunchy goodness!

Vegetable Frittata

Ingredients:

- 3 eggs
- 1/4 cup diced bell peppers
- 1/4 cup diced tomatoes
- 1/4 cup chopped spinach
- Salt and pepper to taste

Instructions:

1. Beat eggs and season with salt and pepper.
2. Pour into a greased oven-safe skillet.
3. Add diced vegetables.
4. Bake at 350°F (175°C) until the frittata is set and lightly golden.

Rice Pudding with Cinnamon

Ingredients:

- 1/2 cup cooked rice
- 1 cup unsweetened almond milk
- 1/2 teaspoon ground cinnamon
- 1 tablespoon honey

Instructions:

1. Combine rice and almond milk in a saucepan.
2. Stir in cinnamon and honey.
3. Simmer until the mixture thickens.
4. Serve warm.

Banana Walnut Pancakes

Ingredients:

- 1 ripe banana, mashed
- 1/2 cup oat flour
- 1/4 cup chopped walnuts
- 1/2 teaspoon baking powder

Instructions:

1. Mix mashed banana, oat flour, walnuts, and baking powder.

2. Cook small pancakes on a non-stick skillet until golden.

Smoothie with Kale and Blueberries

Ingredients:

- 1 cup kale leaves (stems removed)
- 1/2 cup blueberries
- 1/2 cup low-fat yogurt
- 1/2 cup water or almond milk

Instructions:

1. Blend all ingredients until smooth.

2. Enjoy a refreshing and nutritious green smoothie.

Breakfast Burrito with Beans

Ingredients:

- 1 whole wheat tortilla
- 1/4 cup black beans

- 2 scrambled egg whites
- Salsa for topping

Instructions:

1. Lay tortilla flat.
2. Add beans, scrambled egg whites, and salsa.
3. Roll it up into a burrito.

Quinoa Porridge with Almonds

Ingredients:

- 1/2 cup cooked quinoa
- 1/4 cup unsweetened almond milk
- 1/4 cup sliced almonds
- 1/2 teaspoon vanilla extract

Instructions:

1. Combine quinoa, almond milk, sliced almonds, and vanilla extract in a saucepan.
2. Heat gently until warmed through, stirring occasionally.

Greek Yogurt and Fruit Bowl

Ingredients:

- 1/2 cup Greek yogurt
- 1/4 cup mixed fresh fruit (e.g., berries, kiwi)
- 1 tablespoon honey
- 1 tablespoon chopped nuts (e.g., almonds)

Instructions:

1. Place Greek yogurt in a bowl.
2. Top with mixed fresh fruit, honey, and chopped nuts.

Cereal with Fresh Fruit

Ingredients:

- 1/2 cup low-sugar cereal (e.g., bran flakes)
- 1/2 cup unsweetened almond milk
- 1/4 cup sliced fresh fruit (e.g., strawberries, banana)

Instructions:

1. Pour almond milk over cereal.
2. Add sliced fresh fruit for extra flavor and nutrition.

Spinach and Mushroom Omelette

Ingredients:

- 2 eggs
- 1/4 cup sliced mushrooms
- 1/4 cup chopped spinach
- Salt and pepper to taste

Instructions:

1. Beat eggs and season with salt and pepper.
2. In a non-stick pan, sauté mushrooms and spinach.
3. Pour in beaten eggs and cook until set.

Whole Grain Waffles

Ingredients:

- 2 whole grain waffles (store-bought or homemade)
- 1/4 cup low-fat yogurt
- 1/4 cup fresh berries

Instructions:

1. Toast the whole grain waffles until crispy.

2. Serve with a dollop of low-fat yogurt and fresh
   berries.

Avocado Toast with Tomatoes

Ingredients:

- 1 slice whole wheat bread
- 1/2 ripe avocado, mashed
- Sliced cherry tomatoes
- Salt and pepper to taste

Instructions:

1. Toast the whole wheat bread.
2. Spread mashed avocado on top.
3. Add sliced cherry tomatoes and season with salt and
   pepper.

Cottage Cheese and Pineapple

Ingredients:

- 1/2 cup low-fat cottage cheese
- 1/4 cup diced pineapple

Instructions:

1. Place cottage cheese in a bowl.

2. Top with diced pineapple for a sweet and creamy breakfast.

Breakfast Tacos with Salsa

Ingredients:

- 2 small whole wheat tortillas
- 2 scrambled egg whites
- Salsa for topping
- Chopped cilantro (optional)

Instructions:

1. Fill each tortilla with scrambled egg whites.

2. Top with salsa and chopped cilantro if desired.

Sweet Potato Hash

Ingredients:

- 1 cup diced sweet potatoes
- 1/4 cup diced onions
- 1/4 cup bell peppers

- 1/4 cup diced turkey sausage (optional)

Instructions:

1. Sauté sweet potatoes, onions, and bell peppers until tender.
2. Add diced turkey sausage for extra flavor.

Bran Muffins

Ingredients:

- 2 whole grain bran muffins
- 1 tablespoon almond butter (optional)

Instructions:

1. Enjoy whole grain bran muffins as a hearty and fiber-rich breakfast.
2. Spread almond butter on top for added taste.

Chapter 3: Lunch Recipes

In this chapter, we'll explore a variety of lunch recipes that are tailored to support your renal health. These recipes are designed to be both nutritious and satisfying, making your midday meal a delightful experience. Let's dive into these lunchtime creations:

Grilled Chicken Salad

Ingredients:

- 2 boneless, skinless chicken breasts
- Mixed greens
- Cherry tomatoes
- Cucumber slices
- Red onion rings
- Balsamic vinaigrette dressing (low-sodium)

Instructions:

1. Season chicken breasts with salt and pepper.
2. Grill until fully cooked, then slice.

3. Toss mixed greens, tomatoes, cucumbers, and red onion in a bowl.

4. Add grilled chicken on top.

5. Drizzle with balsamic vinaigrette dressing.

Tuna and White Bean Salad

Ingredients:

- Canned tuna in water

- Cannellini beans

- Red onion, finely chopped

- Celery, diced

- Lemon juice

- Olive oil

- Fresh parsley, chopped

Instructions:

1. Drain tuna and beans, then combine in a bowl.

2. Add red onion and celery.

3. In a separate bowl, whisk lemon juice, olive oil, and parsley.

4. Pour dressing over the tuna and bean mixture, toss, and serve.

Quinoa and Vegetable Bowl

Ingredients:

- Quinoa
- Mixed vegetables (bell peppers, zucchini, carrots)
- Olive oil
- Garlic powder
- Lemon juice
- Fresh basil leaves

Instructions:

1. Cook quinoa according to package instructions.
2. Sauté mixed vegetables in olive oil with garlic powder.
3. Combine cooked quinoa and sautéed vegetables.
4. Drizzle with lemon juice and garnish with fresh basil.

Turkey and Avocado Wrap

Ingredients:

- Turkey breast slices
- Whole-grain tortilla wraps
- Avocado slices

- Lettuce
- Dijon mustard

Instructions:

1. Lay out a tortilla wrap.
2. Layer turkey, avocado, lettuce, and a drizzle of Dijon mustard.
3. Roll up the wrap, cut in half, and serve.

Lentil Soup

Ingredients:

- Red lentils
- Carrots, diced
- Celery, chopped
- Onion, finely chopped
- Low-sodium vegetable broth
- Ground cumin
- Ground coriander
- Salt and pepper
- Fresh cilantro, chopped (for garnish)

Instructions:

1. In a large pot, sauté onion, carrots, and celery until soft.
2. Add lentils, vegetable broth, cumin, coriander, salt, and pepper.
3. Simmer until lentils are tender and soup thickens.
4. Garnish with fresh cilantro before serving.

Spinach and Chickpea Salad

Ingredients:

- Baby spinach leaves
- Chickpeas (canned or cooked)
- Cherry tomatoes, halved
- Red onion, thinly sliced
- Feta cheese (optional)
- Balsamic vinaigrette dressing (low-sodium)

Instructions:

1. Combine spinach, chickpeas, cherry tomatoes, and red onion in a bowl.
2. If desired, crumble feta cheese on top.

3. Drizzle with low-sodium balsamic vinaigrette dressing.

Brown Rice and Veggie Stir-fry

Ingredients:

- Brown rice
- Mixed stir-fry vegetables (bell peppers, broccoli, snap peas)
- Low-sodium soy sauce
- Ginger and garlic, minced
- Sesame oil
- Sesame seeds (for garnish)

Instructions:

1. Cook brown rice according to package instructions.
2. In a pan, stir-fry mixed vegetables with ginger and garlic in sesame oil.
3. Add cooked rice and a splash of low-sodium soy sauce.
4. Garnish with sesame seeds.

Salmon Salad with Dill Dressing

Ingredients:

- Grilled or baked salmon fillet
- Mixed greens
- Cucumber slices
- Cherry tomatoes
- Fresh dill
- Greek yogurt (low-fat)
- Lemon juice

Instructions:

1. Flake grilled or baked salmon into bite-sized pieces.
2. Toss mixed greens, cucumber slices, and cherry tomatoes in a bowl.
3. In a separate bowl, mix Greek yogurt, lemon juice, and chopped dill.
4. Add salmon to the salad and drizzle with dill dressing.

Minestrone Soup

Ingredients:

- Low-sodium vegetable broth
- Diced tomatoes (canned)
- Kidney beans (canned)
- Carrots, diced
- Celery, chopped
- Zucchini, sliced
- Whole wheat pasta
- Italian seasoning
- Fresh basil leaves

Instructions:

1. In a pot, combine vegetable broth, diced tomatoes, kidney beans, carrots, celery, and zucchini.
2. Simmer until vegetables are tender.
3. Add whole wheat pasta and Italian seasoning, simmer until pasta is cooked.
4. Garnish with fresh basil before serving.

Shrimp and Broccoli Stir-fry

Ingredients:

- Shrimp, peeled and deveined
- Broccoli florets
- Bell peppers, sliced
- Low-sodium soy sauce
- Garlic and ginger, minced
- Sesame oil
- Cooked brown rice

Instructions:

1. In a pan, stir-fry shrimp, broccoli, and bell peppers with garlic and ginger in sesame oil.
2. Add a splash of low-sodium soy sauce.
3. Serve over cooked brown rice.

Black Bean and Corn Salad

Ingredients:

- Black beans (canned)
- Corn kernels (canned or frozen)
- Red onion, finely chopped

- Red bell pepper, diced

- Fresh cilantro, chopped

- Lime juice

- Olive oil

- Ground cumin

- Salt and pepper

Instructions:

1. Rinse and drain black beans and corn.

2. Combine beans, corn, red onion, and red bell pepper in a bowl.

3. In a separate bowl, whisk together lime juice, olive oil, ground cumin, salt, and pepper.

4. Toss the dressing with the bean and corn mixture, and garnish with fresh cilantro.

Chicken and Rice Bowl

Ingredients:

- Grilled chicken breast, sliced

- Cooked brown rice

- Steamed broccoli florets

- Carrots, julienne

- Teriyaki sauce (low-sodium)

Instructions:

1. Layer sliced grilled chicken, brown rice, steamed broccoli, and julienne carrots in a bowl.
2. Drizzle with low-sodium teriyaki sauce.

Egg Salad Sandwich

Ingredients:

- Hard-boiled eggs, chopped
- Greek yogurt (low-fat)
- Dijon mustard
- Green onions, chopped
- Whole-grain bread

Instructions:

1. In a bowl, combine chopped hard-boiled eggs, Greek yogurt, Dijon mustard, and green onions.
2. Spread the egg salad mixture on whole-grain bread to make a sandwich.

Vegetable and Barley Soup

Ingredients:

- Low-sodium vegetable broth
- Pearl barley
- Mixed vegetables (carrots, celery, peas)
- Onion, chopped
- Garlic, minced
- Bay leaves
- Fresh parsley, chopped

Instructions:

1. In a pot, combine vegetable broth, pearl barley, mixed vegetables, chopped onion, minced garlic, and bay leaves.
2. Simmer until barley is tender and vegetables are cooked.
3. Remove bay leaves, garnish with fresh parsley, and serve.

Caprese Salad

Ingredients:

- Fresh tomatoes, sliced
- Fresh mozzarella cheese, sliced
- Fresh basil leaves
- Balsamic vinegar (low-sodium)
- Olive oil
- Salt and pepper

Instructions:

1. Arrange alternating slices of tomatoes and mozzarella on a plate.
2. Tuck fresh basil leaves between the slices.
3. Drizzle with low-sodium balsamic vinegar and olive oil.
4. Season with a pinch of salt and pepper.

Pita Bread with Hummus

Ingredients:

- Whole wheat pita bread
- Hummus

- Assorted fresh veggies (cucumber, bell peppers, carrots)

Instructions:

1. Cut whole wheat pita bread into wedges.
2. Serve with hummus and assorted fresh veggies for dipping.

Baked Sweet Potato with Beans

Ingredients:

- Sweet potato
- Black beans (canned)
- Salsa
- Greek yogurt (low-fat)
- Fresh cilantro, chopped

Instructions:

1. Bake a sweet potato until tender.
2. Split it open and top with black beans, salsa, a dollop of low-fat Greek yogurt, and fresh cilantro.

Veggie Wrap with Greek Yogurt Sauce

Ingredients:

- Whole-grain tortilla wraps
- Hummus
- Sliced cucumber
- Sliced bell peppers
- Baby spinach leaves
- Greek yogurt sauce (made with low-fat Greek yogurt, lemon juice, and fresh dill)

Instructions:

1. Spread hummus on a whole-grain tortilla wrap.
2. Add cucumber slices, bell peppers, and baby spinach leaves.
3. Drizzle with Greek yogurt sauce.
4. Roll up the wrap and enjoy.

Chapter 4: Dinner Recipes

In this chapter, we embark on a culinary journey through a selection of delightful dinner recipes, each designed to align with a renal-friendly diet. These dishes are not only nourishing but also bursting with flavors that will leave your taste buds craving more. Let's dive into these savory creations that cater to your kidney health.

Baked Salmon with Asparagus

Ingredients:

- 4 salmon fillets
- 1 bunch of fresh asparagus
- Olive oil
- Lemon juice
- Garlic powder
- Salt and pepper to taste

Instructions:

1. Preheat your oven to 400°F (200°C).

2. Place salmon fillets on a baking sheet and season with garlic powder, salt, and pepper.

3. Arrange asparagus around the salmon.

4. Drizzle olive oil and lemon juice over salmon and asparagus.

5. Bake for 15-20 minutes or until salmon flakes easily.

Lemon Herb Grilled Chicken

Ingredients:

- 4 boneless, skinless chicken breasts
- Zest and juice of 2 lemons
- Fresh rosemary and thyme
- Olive oil
- Salt and pepper

Instructions:

1. Mix lemon zest, lemon juice, olive oil, rosemary, and thyme to make a marinade.

2. Marinate chicken breasts for at least 30 minutes.

3. Preheat grill to medium-high heat.

4. Grill chicken for 6-7 minutes per side or until cooked through.

Stuffed Bell Peppers

Ingredients:

- 4 bell peppers (any color)
- 1 cup cooked quinoa
- Lean ground beef or turkey
- Onion, diced
- Tomato sauce
- Italian seasoning
- Grated mozzarella cheese

Instructions:

1. Cut off the tops of the bell peppers and remove seeds.
2. Brown ground meat and onions, then mix with cooked quinoa, tomato sauce, and Italian seasoning.
3. Stuff bell peppers with the mixture and top with mozzarella cheese.
4. Bake at 350°F (175°C) for 25-30 minutes.

Eggplant Parmesan

Ingredients:

- 2 eggplants, sliced

- Bread crumbs

- Egg wash

- Marinara sauce

- Mozzarella cheese

- Parmesan cheese

- Fresh basil

Instructions:

1. Dip eggplant slices in egg wash, then coat with bread crumbs.
2. Bake eggplant slices until crispy.
3. Layer marinara sauce, eggplant, mozzarella, and parmesan cheese.
4. Bake until cheese is bubbly.
5. Garnish with fresh basil.

Beef and Vegetable Stir-fry

Ingredients:

- Lean beef strips

- Assorted vegetables (bell peppers, broccoli, carrots)

- Low-sodium stir-fry sauce

- Garlic and ginger

- Olive oil

Instructions:

1. Heat olive oil in a pan and stir-fry beef until browned. Set aside.
2. In the same pan, stir-fry vegetables with garlic and ginger.
3. Add the beef back to the pan and pour in the stir-fry sauce.
4. Cook until the sauce thickens and coats everything.

Spaghetti Squash with Tomato Sauce

Ingredients:

- Spaghetti squash
- Olive oil
- Garlic
- Canned tomato sauce
- Basil and oregano
- Grated parmesan cheese

Instructions:

1. Cut the spaghetti squash in half and remove seeds.

2. Roast it until the flesh can be easily scraped into "spaghetti" strands.

3. In a separate pan, sauté garlic in olive oil, then add tomato sauce and seasonings.

4. Serve the sauce over the spaghetti squash and top with parmesan.

Teriyaki Tofu and Broccoli

Ingredients:

- Firm tofu, cubed
- Broccoli florets
- Teriyaki sauce (low-sodium)
- Sesame seeds
- Green onions

Instructions:

1. Marinate tofu in teriyaki sauce for at least 30 minutes.

2. Sauté tofu and broccoli until they start to caramelize.

3. Drizzle with more teriyaki sauce and sprinkle with sesame seeds and green onions.

Pork Tenderloin with Apples

Ingredients:

- Pork tenderloin
- Apples, sliced
- Cinnamon and nutmeg
- Low-sodium chicken broth
- Brown sugar (optional)

Instructions:

1. Season pork with cinnamon and nutmeg.
2. Sear pork in a pan until browned, then add apple slices.
3. Pour in chicken broth and simmer until pork is cooked through.
4. Optionally, sprinkle with brown sugar for a touch of sweetness.

Baked Cod with Lemon and Herbs

Ingredients:

- Cod fillets
- Fresh lemon juice and zest
- Fresh herbs (such as thyme and rosemary)
- Olive oil
- Salt and pepper

Instructions:

1. Season cod with lemon juice, zest, herbs, olive oil, salt, and pepper.
2. Bake in a preheated oven at 350°F (175°C) until fish flakes easily.

Quinoa-Stuffed Portobello Mushrooms

Ingredients:

- Portobello mushrooms
- Quinoa
- Spinach
- Feta cheese

- Garlic and onion
- Olive oil

Instructions:

1. Cook quinoa and sauté spinach with garlic and onion.
2. Mix quinoa, spinach, and feta cheese.
3. Stuff portobello mushrooms and bake until tender.

Veggie and Chickpea Curry

Ingredients:

- Chickpeas (canned or cooked)
- Assorted vegetables (e.g., cauliflower, bell peppers)
- Curry paste
- Coconut milk
- Turmeric and cumin
- Fresh cilantro

Instructions:

1. Sauté vegetables in a pan until tender.
2. Add chickpeas, curry paste, coconut milk, and spices.
3. Simmer until flavors meld.

4. Garnish with fresh cilantro.

Turkey Meatloaf

Ingredients:

- Ground turkey
- Oatmeal (as a binder)
- Onions and garlic
- Tomato sauce
- Worcestershire sauce
- Dried thyme and parsley

Instructions:

1. Mix ground turkey, oatmeal, onions, garlic, and seasonings.
2. Shape into a loaf and top with tomato sauce.
3. Bake until cooked through.

Ratatouille

Ingredients:

- Tomatoes, eggplants, zucchini, bell peppers
- Onion and garlic

- Fresh basil and thyme
- Olive oil

Instructions:

1. Sauté onions and garlic in olive oil.
2. Layer sliced vegetables and herbs in a baking dish.
3. Bake until vegetables are tender and flavors meld.

Cilantro Lime Shrimp

Ingredients:

- Shrimp, peeled and deveined
- Fresh cilantro and lime juice
- Garlic
- Olive oil
- Salt and pepper

Instructions:

1. Marinate shrimp in cilantro, lime juice, garlic, olive oil, salt, and pepper.
2. Grill or sauté until shrimp turn pink.

Roasted Vegetable Platter

Ingredients:

- Assorted vegetables (e.g., carrots, broccoli, cauliflower)
- Olive oil
- Garlic and rosemary
- Balsamic vinegar

Instructions:

1. Toss vegetables in olive oil, garlic, and rosemary.
2. Roast until they are caramelized.
3. Drizzle with balsamic vinegar.

Baked Ziti with Ricotta

Ingredients:

- Whole wheat ziti pasta
- Low-fat ricotta cheese
- Marinara sauce
- Mozzarella cheese
- Fresh basil

Instructions:

1. Cook ziti pasta until al dente.
2. Mix with ricotta cheese and marinara sauce.
3. Top with mozzarella cheese and bake until bubbly.
4. Garnish with fresh basil.

BBQ Tofu Skewers

Ingredients:

- Firm tofu, cubed
- BBQ sauce (low-sodium)
- Bell peppers and onions, cut into chunks
- Wooden skewers

Instructions:

1. Marinate tofu in BBQ sauce.
2. Thread tofu, peppers, and onions onto skewers.
3. Grill or bake until tofu is slightly crispy.

Beef and Bean Chili

Ingredients:

- Lean ground beef

- Kidney beans

- Tomatoes and chili powder

- Onion and garlic

- Low-sodium beef broth

Instructions:

1. Brown beef with onions and garlic.

2. Add tomatoes, chili powder, beans, and beef broth.

3. Simmer until flavors meld.

Chapter 5: Snacks and Appetizers

In Chapter 5, we delve into the delightful world of snacks and appetizers that are not only delicious but also kidney-friendly. These recipes are perfect for satisfying those mid-day cravings or impressing guests at gatherings. From creamy dips to crunchy bites, we've got your snacking needs covered.

Guacamole with Veggie Sticks

Ingredients:

- 2 ripe avocados
- 1 small red onion, finely diced
- 2 tomatoes, diced
- 2 cloves garlic, minced
- Juice of 1 lime
- Salt and pepper to taste
- Assorted vegetable sticks (carrots, cucumbers, bell peppers) for dipping

Instructions:

1. Cut the avocados in half, remove the pit, and scoop out the flesh into a bowl.
2. Mash the avocado with a fork until it reaches your desired consistency.
3. Add the diced onion, tomatoes, minced garlic, and lime juice to the mashed avocado. Mix well.
4. Season with salt and pepper to taste.
5. Serve with assorted vegetable sticks for a refreshing and healthy snack.

Mixed Nuts

Ingredients:

*   1 cup mixed unsalted nuts (almonds, cashews, walnuts, etc.)

Instructions:

1. Simply grab a handful of your favorite mixed nuts.
2. Enjoy as a quick and nutritious snack.

Hummus and Whole Wheat Pita

Ingredients:

- Store-bought or homemade hummus
- Whole wheat pita bread, cut into triangles for dipping

Instructions:

1. Scoop a generous portion of hummus into a bowl.
2. Arrange whole wheat pita triangles around the bowl.
3. Dip and savor the creamy goodness of hummus with each bite of pita.

Greek Yogurt Dip with Cucumbers

Ingredients:

- 1 cup Greek yogurt
- 1 cucumber, finely chopped
- 2 tablespoons fresh dill, chopped
- 1 clove garlic, minced
- Salt and pepper to taste

Instructions:

1. In a bowl, combine Greek yogurt, chopped cucumber, fresh dill, and minced garlic.
2. Season with salt and pepper to taste.
3. Mix well and serve as a cool and refreshing dip.

Sliced Apple with Almond Butter

Ingredients:

- Apples, sliced
- Almond butter

Instructions:

1. Slice the apples into thin wedges.
2. Spread almond butter on each apple slice for a delicious and crunchy snack.

Popcorn Seasoned with Herbs

Ingredients:

- 1/2 cup popcorn kernels
- 2 tablespoons olive oil
- 1 teaspoon dried herbs (rosemary, thyme, oregano)

- Salt to taste

Instructions:

1. Pop the popcorn kernels according to package instructions.
2. In a separate bowl, mix the dried herbs and a pinch of salt.
3. Drizzle olive oil over the freshly popped popcorn and toss to coat.
4. Sprinkle the herb mixture over the popcorn and toss again for a savory and aromatic treat.

Cottage Cheese with Peaches

Ingredients:

- Low-fat cottage cheese
- Fresh or canned peaches (in juice, no sugar added)

Instructions:

1. Scoop a portion of low-fat cottage cheese into a bowl.
2. Top it with sliced peaches for a sweet and creamy snack.

Deviled Eggs

Ingredients:

- 6 hard-boiled eggs, peeled and halved
- 2 tablespoons low-fat mayonnaise
- 1 teaspoon Dijon mustard
- Paprika for garnish

Instructions:

1. Carefully remove the egg yolks and place them in a bowl.
2. Mash the yolks with low-fat mayonnaise and Dijon mustard until smooth.
3. Spoon the yolk mixture back into the egg white halves.
4. Sprinkle with paprika for a classic and satisfying appetizer.

Edamame with Sea Salt

Ingredients:

- Edamame pods (frozen or fresh)
- Sea salt

Instructions:

1. Steam or boil the edamame pods until tender.

2. Sprinkle with sea salt and enjoy popping these delicious and protein-packed snacks.

Cherry Tomato Bruschetta

Ingredients:

- Cherry tomatoes, halved

- Fresh basil leaves, chopped

- Balsamic vinegar

- Olive oil

- Whole wheat baguette, sliced and toasted

Instructions:

1. Combine cherry tomatoes and fresh basil in a bowl.

2. Drizzle with balsamic vinegar and olive oil.

3. Spoon the mixture onto toasted whole wheat baguette slices for a flavorful bruschetta.

Trail Mix with Dried Fruit

Ingredients:

- Assorted unsalted nuts (almonds, cashews, etc.)
- Dried fruits (raisins, cranberries, apricots, etc.)

Instructions:

1. Mix your favorite assortment of unsalted nuts and dried fruits in a bowl.
2. Create a custom trail mix that suits your taste preferences, combining the crunch of nuts with the sweetness of dried fruits for a satisfying snack.

Baked Sweet Potato Fries

Ingredients:

- Sweet potatoes, peeled and cut into fries
- Olive oil
- Salt and pepper
- Optional: paprika or garlic powder for added flavor

Instructions:

1. Preheat your oven to 425°F (220°C).

2. Toss sweet potato fries with olive oil, salt, pepper, and any optional seasonings.

3. Spread them on a baking sheet and bake for 20-25 minutes, or until they're crispy and golden brown.

Salsa and Baked Tortilla Chips

Ingredients:

- Whole wheat tortilla wraps

- Olive oil

- Salt

- Store-bought or homemade salsa

Instructions:

1. Preheat your oven to 350°F (175°C).

2. Cut whole wheat tortilla wraps into triangles.

3. Brush them lightly with olive oil and sprinkle with salt.

4. Bake for 10-12 minutes until they become crisp.

5. Serve with your favorite salsa for a satisfying crunch with a zesty kick.

Mini Caprese Skewers

Ingredients:

- Cherry tomatoes
- Fresh mozzarella balls
- Fresh basil leaves
- Balsamic glaze

Instructions:

1. Thread cherry tomatoes, fresh mozzarella balls, and basil leaves onto mini skewers.
2. Drizzle with balsamic glaze for a delightful and elegant appetizer.

Spinach and Artichoke Dip

Ingredients:

- 1 cup cooked spinach, chopped and drained
- 1 cup canned artichoke hearts, chopped and drained
- 1 cup low-fat Greek yogurt
- 1/4 cup grated Parmesan cheese
- 1/4 cup grated low-fat mozzarella cheese
- 1 clove garlic, minced

- Salt and pepper to taste

Instructions:

1. Preheat your oven to 375°F (190°C).
2. In a bowl, combine chopped spinach, artichoke hearts, Greek yogurt, Parmesan cheese, mozzarella cheese, minced garlic, salt, and pepper.
3. Transfer the mixture to a baking dish and bake for about 20 minutes, or until it's bubbly and golden.
4. Serve with whole wheat pita or vegetable sticks for dipping.

Roasted Red Pepper Hummus

Ingredients:

- 1 can (15 ounces) chickpeas, drained and rinsed
- 1/2 cup roasted red peppers, drained
- 2 tablespoons tahini
- 2 cloves garlic, minced
- Juice of 1 lemon
- 2 tablespoons olive oil
- Salt and pepper to taste

Instructions:

1. In a food processor, combine chickpeas, roasted red peppers, tahini, minced garlic, lemon juice, and olive oil.

2. Blend until smooth and creamy.

3. Season with salt and pepper to taste.

4. Serve with vegetable sticks or whole wheat pita for dipping.

Stuffed Mushrooms

Ingredients:

- Large white mushrooms
- Low-fat cream cheese
- Fresh parsley, chopped
- Garlic powder
- Paprika

Instructions:

1. Remove the stems from the mushrooms and clean them.

2. In a bowl, mix low-fat cream cheese with chopped fresh parsley, a pinch of garlic powder, and paprika.

3. Stuff each mushroom cap with the cream cheese mixture.

4. Bake in a preheated oven at 375°F (190°C) for 15-20 minutes or until mushrooms are tender and filling is lightly golden.

Avocado Slices with Lime

Ingredients:

- Ripe avocados
- Fresh lime juice

Instructions:

1. Slice ripe avocados into thin wedges.
2. Drizzle with fresh lime juice to enhance the flavor and prevent browning.
3. Enjoy this simple, nutritious, and refreshing snack.

Chapter 6: Desserts

When it comes to satisfying your sweet tooth while following a renal diet, Chapter 6 has you covered with an array of delightful desserts that won't compromise your kidney health. These desserts are not only kidney-friendly but also packed with flavor. Let's dive into these delectable treats:

Baked Apples with Cinnamon

Ingredients:

- 4 apples
- 2 tablespoons cinnamon
- 1 tablespoon honey (optional)

Instructions:

1. Preheat your oven to 350°F (175°C).
2. Core the apples and place them in a baking dish.
3. Sprinkle cinnamon over each apple and drizzle with honey if desired.

4. Bake for 30-40 minutes until the apples are tender.
   Serve warm.

Berry Parfait with Greek Yogurt

Ingredients:

- 1 cup Greek yogurt
- 1 cup mixed berries (strawberries, blueberries, raspberries)
- 2 tablespoons honey (optional)
- 1/4 cup granola

Instructions:

1. In a glass or bowl, layer Greek yogurt, mixed berries, and granola.
2. Drizzle honey on top for sweetness if desired.
3. Repeat the layers.
4. Finish with a sprinkle of granola on top.

Chocolate Avocado Mousse

Ingredients:

- 2 ripe avocados

- 1/4 cup cocoa powder

- 1/4 cup honey (adjust to taste)

- 1 teaspoon vanilla extract

Instructions:

1. Blend avocados, cocoa powder, honey, and vanilla extract until smooth.

2. Refrigerate for at least 30 minutes before serving.

Rice Pudding with Raisins

Ingredients:

- 1 cup cooked white rice

- 1 cup milk (or milk substitute)

- 1/4 cup raisins

- 1/4 teaspoon ground cinnamon

Instructions:

1. In a saucepan, combine cooked rice and milk.

2. Cook over low heat, stirring, until thickened.

3. Stir in raisins and cinnamon.

4. Let it cool before serving.

Banana Ice Cream

Ingredients:

- 4 ripe bananas, frozen
- 1 teaspoon vanilla extract

Instructions:

1. Blend frozen bananas and vanilla extract until creamy.
2. Serve immediately as a healthy ice cream alternative.

Lemon Sorbet

Ingredients:

- 1 cup freshly squeezed lemon juice
- 1 cup water
- 1/2 cup sugar (or sweetener of choice)

Instructions:

1. Mix lemon juice, water, and sugar until sugar dissolves.
2. Freeze the mixture in a shallow dish, stirring every 30 minutes, until it reaches a sorbet consistency.

Peach and Berry Crisp

Ingredients:

- 2 cups sliced peaches (fresh or canned in juice)
- 1 cup mixed berries (strawberries, blueberries, raspberries)
- 1/2 cup rolled oats
- 1/4 cup almond meal
- 2 tablespoons honey
- 1/2 teaspoon cinnamon

Instructions:

1. Preheat your oven to 350°F (175°C).
2. In a bowl, combine peaches, mixed berries, and half of the honey. Mix gently.
3. In another bowl, combine oats, almond meal, remaining honey, and cinnamon.
4. Place the fruit mixture in a baking dish and top with the oat mixture.
5. Bake for 25-30 minutes or until the topping is golden brown.

Oatmeal Cookies with Raisins

Ingredients:

- 1 cup rolled oats
- 1/2 cup mashed bananas
- 1/4 cup raisins
- 1/4 cup unsweetened applesauce
- 1/2 teaspoon cinnamon

Instructions:

1. Preheat your oven to 350°F (175°C).
2. In a bowl, combine oats, mashed bananas, raisins, applesauce, and cinnamon.
3. Drop spoonfuls of the mixture onto a baking sheet.
4. Bake for 15-20 minutes until the cookies are firm and lightly browned.

Angel Food Cake with Berries

Ingredients:

- 1 store-bought angel food cake
- 2 cups mixed berries (strawberries, blueberries, raspberries)

- 1/2 cup whipped cream (optional)

Instructions:

1. Slice the angel food cake into serving portions.
2. Top each slice with a generous serving of mixed berries.
3. Add a dollop of whipped cream if desired.

Pumpkin Pie with Oat Crust

Ingredients:

- 1 pre-made oat crust (store-bought or homemade)
- 1 can (15 ounces) pumpkin puree
- 1/2 cup milk (or milk substitute)
- 1/4 cup honey
- 1 teaspoon pumpkin pie spice

Instructions:

1. Preheat your oven to 350°F (175°C).
2. In a bowl, mix pumpkin puree, milk, honey, and pumpkin pie spice.
3. Pour the mixture into the oat crust.
4. Bake for 35-40 minutes or until the pie is set.

5. Allow it to cool before slicing.

Frozen Yogurt with Mango

Ingredients:

- 1 cup plain yogurt (low-fat or non-fat)
- 1 ripe mango, peeled and diced
- 2 tablespoons honey (adjust to taste)
- 1/2 teaspoon vanilla extract

Instructions:

1. Blend plain yogurt, diced mango, honey, and vanilla extract until smooth.
2. Pour the mixture into an ice cream maker and follow the manufacturer's instructions.
3. Once churned, transfer to a container and freeze for a firmer consistency.

Chia Seed Pudding

Ingredients:

- 1/4 cup chia seeds
- 1 cup milk (or milk substitute)

- 1 tablespoon honey

- 1/2 teaspoon vanilla extract

- Fresh berries for topping

Instructions:

1. In a bowl, combine chia seeds, milk, honey, and vanilla extract.

2. Stir well and refrigerate for at least 2 hours or overnight.

3. Serve with fresh berries on top.

Poached Pears in Red Wine

Ingredients:

- 4 pears, peeled and cored

- 1 bottle red wine

- 1/2 cup sugar (or sweetener of choice)

- 1 cinnamon stick

- 4 cloves

- 1 strip of orange zest

Instructions:

1. In a large saucepan, combine red wine, sugar, cinnamon stick, cloves, and orange zest.

2. Bring to a simmer and add the pears.

3. Poach the pears for about 20-30 minutes until tender.

4. Remove the pears and let the syrup reduce until thickened.

5. Drizzle the syrup over the poached pears before serving.

Almond and Cherry Biscotti

Ingredients:

- 1 cup almond flour
- 1/2 cup dried cherries
- 1/4 cup honey
- 1 teaspoon almond extract

Instructions:

1. Preheat your oven to 350°F (175°C).

2. In a bowl, combine almond flour, dried cherries, honey, and almond extract.

3. Form the dough into a log shape on a baking sheet.

4. Bake for 20-25 minutes until firm and slightly golden.

5. Allow it to cool, then slice into biscotti-sized pieces.

Carrot Cake Bites

Ingredients:

- 1 cup shredded carrots
- 1/2 cup rolled oats
- 1/4 cup chopped walnuts
- 1/4 cup honey
- 1/2 teaspoon cinnamon
- 1/4 teaspoon nutmeg

Instructions:

1. In a food processor, blend shredded carrots, rolled oats, chopped walnuts, honey, cinnamon, and nutmeg.

2. Roll the mixture into bite-sized balls.

3. Refrigerate for 30 minutes before serving.

Pineapple Sorbet

Ingredients:

- 2 cups frozen pineapple chunks
- 1/4 cup coconut milk
- 1 tablespoon honey (adjust to taste)

Instructions:

1. Blend frozen pineapple chunks, coconut milk, and honey until smooth.
2. Serve immediately for a refreshing treat.

Fig and Walnut Bars

Ingredients:

- 1 cup dried figs
- 1/2 cup walnuts
- 1/4 cup almond meal
- 1/4 cup honey
- 1/2 teaspoon vanilla extract

Instructions:

1. In a food processor, combine dried figs, walnuts, almond meal, honey, and vanilla extract.
2. Blend until the mixture forms a dough-like consistency.
3. Press the mixture into a square pan and refrigerate until set.
4. Cut into bars and enjoy.

Chocolate-Dipped Strawberries

Ingredients:

- 12 fresh strawberries
- 1/4 cup dark chocolate chips
- 1/2 teaspoon coconut oil (optional)

Instructions:

1. Wash and dry the strawberries.
2. Melt dark chocolate chips (and coconut oil, if using) in a microwave or double boiler.
3. Dip each strawberry into the melted chocolate, allowing excess to drip off.

4. Place them on a parchment-lined tray and refrigerate until the chocolate hardens.

CONCLUSION

As you reach the conclusion of this guide, it's important to remember that a renal diet isn't just a temporary fix but a lifelong commitment to your kidney health. Let's take a moment to reflect on some key takeaways:

1. Sustainability: The renal diet isn't a crash diet; it's a sustainable way of eating that can help protect your kidneys and overall health for years to come. Embrace it as a lifestyle choice.

2. Knowledge is Power: You've armed yourself with valuable knowledge about foods, nutrients, and cooking techniques that support kidney health. Keep learning and staying informed.

3. Small Steps Matter: Making gradual changes to your diet and lifestyle can lead to big improvements in your kidney health. Don't be discouraged by setbacks; focus on progress.

4. Hydration Matters: Adequate hydration is essential for kidney function. Keep track of your fluid intake

and discuss with your healthcare provider how much is right for you.

5. Stay Positive: Maintaining a renal diet can be challenging, but a positive attitude and a support system of friends and family can make all the difference.

6. Adapt and Thrive: Life is full of changes, and your dietary needs may evolve. Be prepared to adapt and thrive as you continue your journey to optimal kidney health.

As you conclude your exploration of the renal diet, know that you have the tools and knowledge to make informed choices about what you eat and how you care for your kidneys. This chapter marks the beginning of a new phase in your life—a healthier, kidney-conscious one. Keep moving forward with confidence and commitment, and may your path be paved with good health and well-being.

9 798864 001516